Giselle Roeder

Healing with Water

Kneipp Hydrotherapy at home

alive books

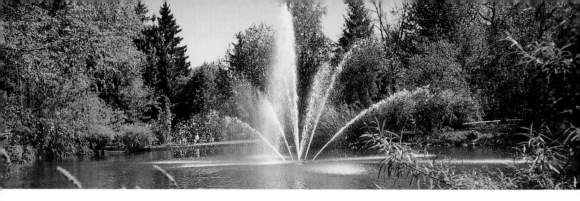

Contents

All About Healing with Water

Note: Conversions in this book (from imperial to metric) are not exact. They have been rounded to the nearest measurement for convenience. Exact measurements are given in imperial. The recipes in this book are by no means to be taken as therapeutic. They simply promote the philosophy of both the author and *alive* books in relation to whole foods, health and nutrition, while incorporating the practical advice given by the author in the first section of the book.

Recipes

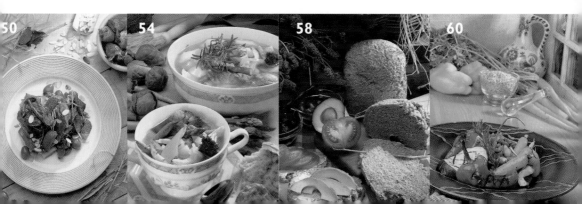

50 54 58 60

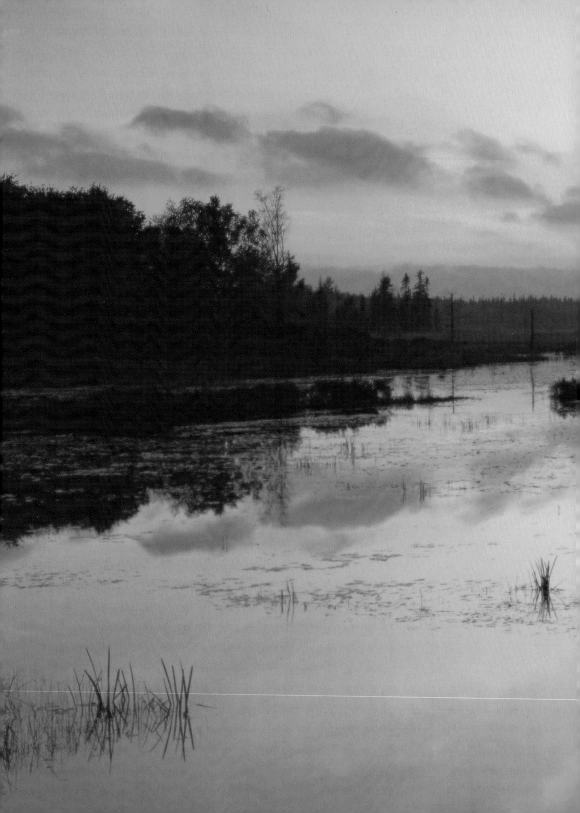

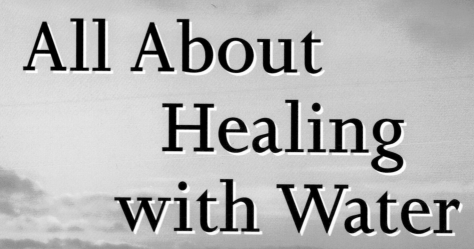

All About Healing with Water

One might argue that hydrotherapy is even more important today than it was in Father Kneipp's time.

Introduction . . . .

Water is life, and for centuries, people have been drawn to the Earth's springs to revitalize themselves. During the 19th century, Father Sebastian Kneipp recognized the value of water for regenerating the tired and sick body, and developed a system that you can easily use at home in the 21st century to do the following:

- relieve stress
- improve circulation
- build immunity
- feel young and vital
- relieve headaches
- ease arthritis
- correct digestive problems
- help you sleep
- revitalize your sex life

One might argue that hydrotherapy is even more important today than it was in Kneipp's time! But Kneipp therapy is so much more than just taking the right kind of bath. Kneipp developed a whole body-and-mind philosophy for a balanced life. His "five pillars" include water therapy, nature's apothecary, food as medicine, "he who rests, rusts," and spiritual harmony. He sought a balance of all the elements of one's life. It would seem we need his wisdom now more than ever.

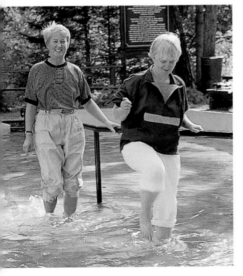

Get Your Feet Wet! . . . .

When I was twenty-three, I developed circulation problems. After months of conventional medication, my medical doctor sent me to undergo the "Kneipp cure." I had no idea what that entailed, but I learned! I literally got my feet wet. I learned that Kneipp was the famous Water Doctor, a 19th-century Bavarian priest who had transformed the sleepy village of Wörishofen into a world-renowned spa.

But you don't have to go to a European spa to benefit from Kneipp's wisdom. You can use his water therapy techniques at home in your own bathroom. In combination with his other principles for a balanced, healthful life, water therapy can help you achieve good health. As more and more drugs flood the market, offering to cure any and all ailments without regard to side effects, it is more important than ever to know how pure, simple water can help to restore your health.

The Founding Father ......

Sebastian Kneipp (1821-1897), a poor weaver's son, developed tuberculosis at an early age. When Sebastian spit up blood, his father simply said, "all weavers spit blood." There was no treatment, but Sebastian was determined to get well and follow his dream of one day becoming a priest. Luck placed in his hands an old book about healing with water, written by a father and son team of doctors in the 18th century. He followed the advice faithfully and eventually got well.

To rinse out impurities, he drank lots of fresh water. He also rubbed his chest with cold water. His biggest problem was finding a private spot where he could immerse his whole body in the cold water of a river several times a week, so he started using a watering can to douse himself. He soon began to feel better.

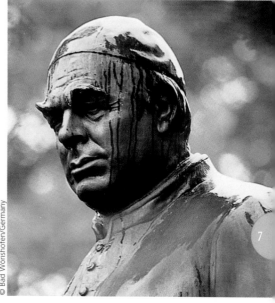

Father Kneipp (1821-1897).

Sebastian started to treat other students, with the same good results. Finally, he passed a rigid health test in 1852 and was declared fit to be ordained. His dream to serve God was fulfilled. But he couldn't refrain from helping the poor villagers with their health concerns. At odds with the church, the pharmacists and the medical profession, his life became a nightmare, but he couldn't stop himself from helping those who needed it.

Father Kneipp eventually developed the original water cure into a system of full or partial bath immersions with herbal extracts added, effusions, alternating temperatures, washings, wraps, steam and ice, and introduced the use of clay and cottage cheese for healing. He collected, experimented with, and cataloged hundreds of herbs. He promoted simple, down-to-earth food, physical work and exercise, and even maintained to the idle rich that work is a form of prayer. He realized that most disease was related directly to emotional distress.

Kneipp's deep trust in God and the power of nature, coupled with his tremendous perception and the gift of healing, helped him to diagnose problems and offer the right treatment. His success rate was unequalled.

Finally, to keep the help-seeking people from all over Europe at bay, Kneipp wrote a book entitled My Water Cure. This book sold as many copies as the Bible at the time, was used in just about every household, and was translated into seventeen languages. He became known as the Water Doctor.

Driven to Help and Heal

Eventually, Kneipp was called to Rome, where the Pope said to him, "so you are driven to heal; you cannot help it?" Kneipp, anticipating his excommunication from the church, very unhappily did not deny this. But the Pope gave him his blessing. This opened the floodgates to an ever-increasing number of health seekers coming to his home village, Wörishofen. The wealthy, aristocrats, the royalty of Europe, even a maharajah of India came to him. Medical doctors wanted to learn Kneipp's techniques and entrepreneurs invested in hotels and bathhouses in Wörishofen. The guest lists read like a Who's Who.

The village of Wörishofen remains a destination for health seekers today, where many establishments are health-driven, such as this beautiful spot where fresh juices and whole foods are served.

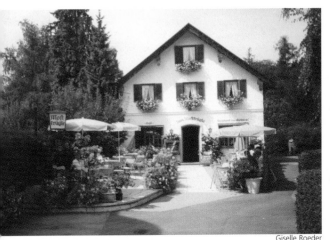

Giselle Roeder

Father Kneipp wrote two more books, *This Is How Thou Shall Live* and *My Testament and Codicil*, in which he challenges the medical profession to adopt his system, develop it further, and "make it accessible to all people." Today, more than a century after Kneipp's death, the Kneipp water cure is alive and well. Hundreds of Kneipp spa cities cater to millions of people all over the world.

In Europe, mainly Germany,

insurance companies pay for the cost of a Kneipp water cure to prevent disease and speed recovery after an operation, heart attack or nervous breakdown. A clinical study in Austria proved a threefold reduction in health-care costs when the Kneipp cure was used to complement conventional treatments. Through a man named Benedict Lust, whom Kneipp cured of tuberculosis, the Kneipp cure came to North America, where it is one of the theories behind naturopathy.

What Can Water Do? . . . . . .

The Kneipp System, and water therapy in particular, can do many things for you. You want to feel fit, strong and full of pep and energy, and by using Kneipp's principles on a daily basis, you can. Hot water drains energy, lowers blood pressure and removes your skin's natural oils, leaving it dry. Warm water on a daily basis ages you faster. But if you use cold water after the warm water, it will normalize all body functions.

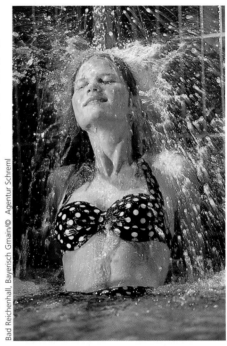

Bad Reichenhall, Bayerisch Gmain/© Agentur Schreml

The change between warm and cold stabilizes your heart function and strengthens your respiratory system, allowing more oxygen to be taken in, so you feel fit and your energy level increases. You might not like it at first, but in time you will get used to it. In fact, you will miss it when you don't have time to do it!

A full-body warm-cold treatment (such as a shower) should not be done in the evening before going to bed, but it is a great pick-me-up when you come home exhausted and have to go out again; otherwise it is a morning exercise. Do it regularly, and you'll see an improvement in your health in a very short time. In addition to remedying some specific problems, which we'll look at a little later, water therapy can do the following:

Build immunity: The change between hot and cold water, used regularly, will cause your body to build more disease-fighting cells. Once your body is stronger it will be able to fight colds

A clinical study in Austria proved a threefold reduction in health-care costs when the Kneipp cure was used to complement conventional treatments.

9

and flu, as well as other maladies, much more effectively.

Improve circulation: The movement of the blood in the body is like the gasoline in a car: Nothing works without it. If the circulation is strong, you won't have any problems. If the circulation is weak, cold hands and feet are just the first health changes you will notice. Spider veins, and so-called "broken" veins in the facial skin, tell the story. Next you will notice varicose veins, and these can lead to more serious problems. Kneipp's system of hot and cold rinses, baths, wraps and other treatments definitely improves circulation.

Help you feel young longer: The hormone system changes as the years go by, but as long as the body's functions are in tune with each other, you will feel young. For example, if the thyroid gland either over- or under-functions, a number of other systems are affected. You might feel unusually tired, or you might have unexplained weight loss or gain, headaches or insomnia. These ailments will affect your feeling of well being and you will

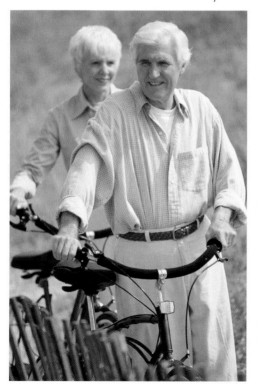

age faster. Good circulation is a prerequisite to keep everything functioning. Using Kneipp therapy to help it along is definitely the easiest answer.

Help you enjoy your "golden years": With a fit and functioning body there is absolutely no reason to feel old when you celebrate your sixty-fifth birthday! Now is the time to do all the things you never had time for, enroll in some courses, learn Tai Chi or Scottish dancing, travel and make new friends. I can assure you from my own experience of a lifetime of living with the Kneipp System that my body functions just as it did twenty years ago. Sure, there is a little rust here and there, but that is no reason to worry.

What Is Water Therapy, Anyway?

You could be using water therapy right now without even being aware that that's what it is! A simple and relaxing soak in the tub is water therapy! The Kneipp System symbol is a watering can. In the beginning it was used to administer rinses: full body, up to the knee, up to or including the hips, the arms, the shoulders and the back. Kneipp developed a technique that is used to this day, though the watering can has been replaced with a hose. The pressure of the water coming out of the hose should be such that it springs up about one hand width high when the hose is held up. The hose's diameter is slightly wider than that of a garden hose. The hose should be held in such a way that the water covers the skin like a mantle, without air trapped underneath or within the water. It is important that the water coat the body evenly without splashing over the skin.

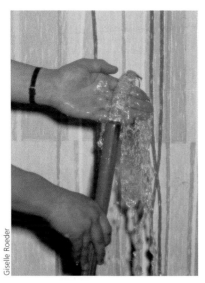

Giselle Roeder

A showerhead with a five-foot hose enables you to direct the water where you want it without having to move your body around.

All rinses start at the farthest spot from the heart; for example, on the baby toe of the right foot for lower-body treatments and on the little finger of the right hand for the upper body. The hose is moved slowly and evenly up the leg or arm, always making sure that the water covers the whole body part. The water stops just above the knee, hip, shoulder or whichever part the treatment is concentrating on, before it is moved down again.

First the water is moved upward on the outside of the leg or arm, then down on the inside. Comfortably hot water is used for an alternating-temperature treatment until the skin glows, followed by approximately fifteen to twenty seconds of cold water. A second hot rinse is used, and then the treatment is finished with a cold rinse.

The soles of the feet are rinsed last, first the right one and then the left. The water should just be wiped off by hand, although I recommend a towel for the soles of the feet and between the toes. Put on thick socks and go for a brisk walk or back to bed, depending on what the doctor ordered.

Some cautions for water treatments:
- It is crucial to stay warm.
- Do not apply a cold treatment to a cold body.
- No treatment should be performed in a cold room.
- Do not apply a treatment with a full or empty stomach.
- Two opposite treatments (for example, arms and legs) should not be performed within a short time.

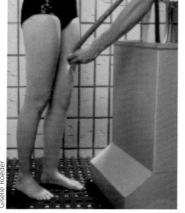

All rinses start at the farthest spot from the heart and move slowly and evenly up the leg or arm.

All rinses on the lower body are done as described above, except the full lower-body rinse. This treatment includes a spiral around the tummy at the final cold rinse before moving the water down the left leg. Lower-body rinses are recommended for poor circulation, headaches, low blood pressure, swelling, water retention, vein problems, nervousness and insomnia.

For upper-body rinses the patient bends down over a divider, such as a chair or the edge of the bathtub. The arm or shoulder rinse is straightforward. For the chest rinse the hose is held under the bent-over body and the water is moved in a figure eight over the chest. Upper-body rinses, depending on the use of cold, warm or alternating cold and warm water, are for unusual tiredness, muscle tension, high blood pressure, improving immunity, tissue toning and a weak heart. Those with chronic or coronary heart problems and asthma should not have this treatment.

One more rinse is done with the hose: the "blitz." Using a high-pressure attachment (which is not readily available for home use), the water is moved over the body with whip-like massage motions. Only fit and strong individuals can experience this deep-tissue treatment.

Complementary—Not Alternative . . . .

To call Kneipp Hydrotherapy "alternative" would mean using water to cure a disease just with this method. This would not be a realistic expectation. However, using a conventional medical treatment and complementing it with water therapy has produced incredible results. A large Austrian hospital carried out an experiment: One group of patients was treated just with conventional methods, while a second group received the same treatments plus water therapy. The result was that the second group got well much faster. Another important result was that the cost of treatment went down considerably.

Kneipp Hydrotherapy, used as a complementary method in hospital settings for acute cases or in sanatoriums or recovery homes for convalescence after surgery or serious illness, not only helps the patient back to health faster, it saves the medical system money.

The Europeans have made water treatment into an art form, saving health-insurance companies bundles of money through prevention and rehabilitation.

The Spa

Spas have always been associated with water. Five thousand years ago, the Chinese, Persians, Indians and Egyptians used water for healing. Later, the Greeks and Romans developed bath methods as part of their cultures. A new bath boom flourished in the 16th and 17th centuries. Now that the excitement over chemical based wonder drugs has worn off, cries of "back to nature" can be heard as we search for alternatives. Renowned healers (Hippocrates, Paracelsus, Floyer, Priessnitz, Hufeland and Kneipp) have brought water therapy to us.

One of the nicest things you can do for yourself is take a spa holiday. The ambience, the pampering, the relaxation, all allow for a reunification of body and soul. The feeling of being "whole" again can be wonderful. In North America, the word "spa" conjures up images of beauty treatments—facials, massages, manicures, weight-loss programs and exercise. In Europe, the concept is totally different.

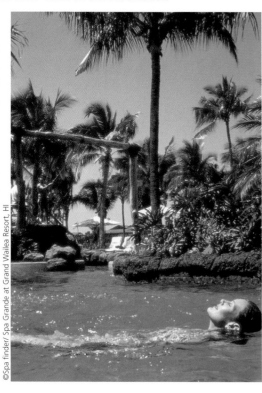

©Spa finder/ Spa Grande at Grand Wailea Resort, HI

13

These elements are frills to a spa vacation. For centuries, Europeans have used spas for the improvement of health, youth and vigor, as well as for socializing.

A spa means thermal or mineral water treatments; the water is used as it comes from the Earth. In North America, hot springs are harnessed in large swimming pools and are open to everyone. In Europe, the water is pumped into "cure houses," with access available only with a doctor's prescription. It is used to ease the pain of rheumatism or arthritis; increase circulation; improve the respiratory, hormonal or immune systems; help skin diseases and many more ailments.

The Europeans have developed water treatment into an art form, saving health-insurance companies bundles of money. The emphasis is on prevention of diseases and on rehabilitation after breakdowns in health.

The Hot Tub

We have all seen hot tubs and whirlpools in recreational centers, on cruise ships, beside swimming pools or even in some homes. Sometimes you will see a warning: "Do not use pool longer than 10 minutes." Hardly anybody follows this advice—I know people who sit for an hour in the very hot water. Besides removing the natural oils from the skin (just look at your fingertips: they shrivel up!), the blood pressure might sink to a dangerously low level and fainting or even a stroke could result. If you do use overly hot water to relax (for sure, hot water and the resulting drop in blood pressure do relax you) get out as soon as you feel your head becoming hot or sweaty. Watch the skin on your fingertips; as soon as it starts to look whitish and form vertical lines, it is time to have a cold rinse. Be sure to rinse from the feet up and not like a shower from the head down. I will describe specific methods later.

The German Kur

In Germany, where Kneipp Hydrotherapy was born, insurance companies pay for a so-called Kur (cure)—a stay in one of the hundreds of Kneipp spa cities—if a medical doctor prescribes it. The insurance companies know that it is less expensive to pay for three or four weeks of treatment at the spa before a nervous breakdown or a heart attack than to pay to repair the damage to the patient once it has been done. Spa treatments are part of a medical system aimed at prevention and recuperation. The Kur is purely for medical reasons.

What happens at the spa? After a thorough examination by a registered Kneipp doctor, you are given a "cure book" with the recommended treatments for each day of the first week. After every treatment, which consists of body wraps, washings, rinses or bathing, you go back to bed for approximately half to one hour. During the second, third and fourth weeks, you again visit the doctor, and the treatments for that week are written into your book.

Kneipp Hydrotherapy at Home . . . .

To know Kneipp Hydrotherapy is to have the knowledge to use water to influence your body's systems. You will use warm water, cold water, alternate temperatures, steam, ice, water in bathtubs or as rinses and showers, water with or without pressure, and water in wraps and as washings for the whole body, or for specific parts of it.

Kneipp Hydrotherapy does not require special mineral or thermal water; the water you get through your faucets is fine.

Your Bathroom Is Your Health Spa

Learn and enjoy Kneipp Hydrotherapy at home! You have a bathtub. You have a shower. You have a sink—maybe even two. Hot and cold water is available. You are equipped! If your showerhead is attached to the wall, unscrew it and attach a five-foot hose with a new showerhead. This enables you to take the shower off the wall and direct the water where you want it without moving your body. The new showerhead may even have different settings for the pressure of the water. Buy a little kitchen timer to time your treatments. You might want to get a bathtub mat that will allow you to stand a little above the water.

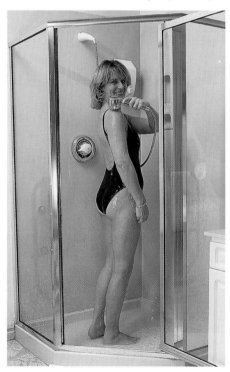

The Morning Shower

Do what you always do: Set the temperature to your liking and use

Since no special water or equipment is required, you can easily do Kneipp Hydrotherapy treatments at home to prevent problems, increase your immunity and circulation, and become a healthier person.

your favorite shower gel or soap for your cleansing routine and rinse well. Then take the shower off the hook, set the temperature to temperate or cold, take a deep breath and, while exhaling, direct the water starting from your right baby toe, up the outside of the leg and over the hip. Quickly move the water down on the inside of the leg, all the while making sure that the water covers the skin like a mantle—it should not splash too much. Now move the water over to the left baby toe and do the same: Up the outside of the leg, down on the inside.

If you feel like it, you can repeat this procedure with warm or hot water and after that, once again, do a quick cold rinse. Make sure you are not standing in the cold water; stand with your legs apart so that the water runs down the middle of the bathtub. I usually rinse the bathtub with hot water after my cold rinse.

The change in water temperature will increase circulation to the lower extremities but release pressure or congestion in the upper body and head. Dry yourself and get dressed. If you have the time, wrap yourself in a big towel or warm housecoat and go back to bed for fifteen to twenty minutes without drying off (except for your face, between legs and toes).

After a few weeks of this treatment, change it as follows: Instead of moving the cold water just to your hips, move it to your right hand and from there up to the shoulder. Let part of it run over your back and part over your chest. Go up on the outside of the arm and down on the inside. Do the same on the left side. Once you get used to the procedure and dare a bit more, bend forward and move the water in a figure eight over your chest before moving it down again.

These treatments can become a daily routine. They will enhance your immune system and protect you better from colds and flu. Choose one type of treatment per morning; don't try to do them all! Remember to keep breathing: Exhale as you move the cold water up your body; inhale when you are moving it down toward the toes.

Never read or watch TV when resting after a treatment. Direct your mind toward the area treated or just let your thoughts drift. I always put on warm socks to make sure my feet don't get cold. Staying warm is a key to the Kneipp System.

Upper-Body Rinses

Upper-body rinses are effective for toning skin and relieving tension.

Facial or beauty rinse: This rinse is done with cold water only, and can be done several times a day. To protect clothing, wrap a towel around your neck. Bend over the bathtub. Starting on the right side, move the water back and forth across your forehead, up and down your cheeks, and finish by circling your face three times.

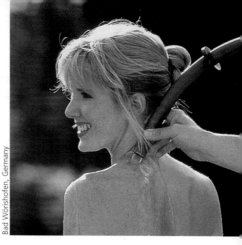

Pat the skin dry and massage it with your favorite lotion or cream. This treatment increases skin tone, is refreshing and has a stimulating effect when you are tired, nervous or have a headache. Do not use it if you have serious eye problems.

Hot shoulder/back rinse: If you have tension in your shoulders or your back, let hot water run over the area for several minutes. Pat your feet dry and wrap yourself in a warm housecoat and go back to bed.

Cold or alternating-temperature arm or shoulder rinse: For the cold treatment, bend over your bathtub, take your showerhead off the hook, set the temperature and move the flowing water up the arm to the shoulder, starting with the right hand. Let the water run down from the shoulder for a few seconds, then move down. Repeat on the left side. Don't do any cold treatments if your hands are cold!

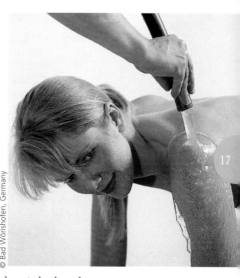

For the alternating-temperature treatment, do as above, but start with warm water. Let it run over your arm and/or shoulder until the skin glows, showing an increase in circulation. Move down, then do the left side. Set the water temperature to cold and repeat. Alternating-temperature treatments are repeated twice: warm-cold, warm-cold.

Arm rinses are refreshing, increase circulation and are prescribed for a nervous heart, low blood pressure or general tiredness.

Cold or alternating-temperature breast rinse: For the cold rinse, start on the right hand and move the water up to the shoulder and down again. Do the left arm. Now take the water up the right inner arm to the chest, do a figure eight around both breasts, and go down on the inner left arm. For the alternating-temperature treatment, do as above, starting with the warm water. After both arms are done, do the breasts as described above.

Finish by going down the inner left arm. Change temperature to cold and do the cold rinse as above. Change to warm again and repeat. Finish with a cold application. Breast rinses are refreshing and healing for general tiredness, increased circulation and improved immunity; they also tighten the breast tissue.

Lower-body Rinses

Among the many benefits gained with lower-body rinses is the relief of menopause symptoms and the increase in libido.

Cold or alternating-temperature knee rinse: Do the cold rinse only if your feet are warm. Stand in the bathtub, either with your legs wide apart to avoid the flowing water in the middle, or on a grate at least an inch high to let the water run underneath. Take the shower in your right hand, and starting on the baby toe of the right foot, direct the water up the outside of the leg to just above the knee.

Move the water two or three times back and forth before moving it down on the inside of the leg; repeat on the left side.

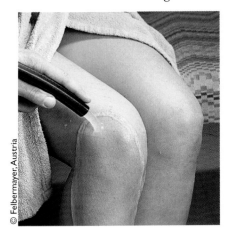

Lift the right foot and move the water over the sole of the foot; repeat on the left.

Step out of the bathtub, dry the soles of your feet and between the toes, put warm socks on and either go to bed or for a brisk walk. Never sit down after a foot or leg treatment! Move!

For the alternating-temperature treatment, start with warm water. First do the right leg, then the left. Do the same with the cold water. Repeat the warm treatment, then finish with cold. At the end, do the soles of your feet—first the right, then the left.

Alternating-temperature and cold knee rinses are effective for tension headaches, circulation problems in the legs, hot flashes during menopause, insomnia and high blood pressure. Do not use during menstruation, or if you have a bladder infection, sciatica pain or bad varicose veins.

Cold or alternating-temperature hip rinse: This treatment is basically the same as the knee rinse, except that you move the water up to just above the hipbone. The final cold rinse can include a spiral around the abdomen. Start on the lower right of your abdomen, where your appendix is (or was) and move two or three times around the abdomen before going down on the left inner leg. Finish with the soles of your feet. This treatment is especially effective for the symptoms of menopause.

Washings

Washings are the mildest of all Kneipp treatments. They are done with a folded linen towel using either cold or temperate water. Vinegar, salt or herbal tea can be added. Cold water and vinegar will increase skin metabolism, promote perspiration and will release toxins. The skin is the "third kidney!"

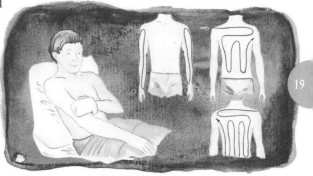

Upper-body washing technique.

Washing can be done on the whole body, on the upper or lower body or just on the abdomen. The best time to do it is in the early morning; you can do it sitting in or on your bed. A moist film should remain on the skin and slowly evaporate while you lie covered in bed. The treatment is never done on a cold body, and should be done quickly to avoid cooling your sleep-warm body. Without drying off, slip back into your pajamas or gown and cuddle back into bed. Most likely you will have another deep sleep.

Full or partial washings will help to stabilize the nervous system, improve circulation, build immunity, increase your metabolism and ease chronic rheumatic problems.

Upper-body washing: Wrap a wet towel around your hand and move it quickly up on the outside of the right arm and down on

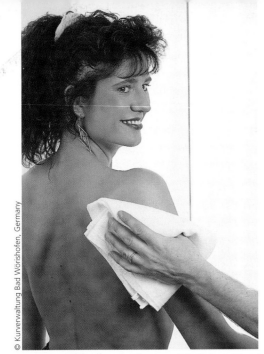

the inside; include the underarm area. Do the left arm, chest and back. Put your pajama top back on and cuddle under the blanket. Do not dry!

Lower-body washing: This is basically the same as the upper-body washing. Start on the right foot, and go up the leg. Do the left side, then do the abdomen in a spiral. Go back to bed and stay warm.

Full-body washing: Combine the upper- and lower-body washings. Start with the right arm, then do the left arm, chest, neck, abdomen and back. Now wash the lower body starting on the right foot; then do the right leg, left foot and left leg. Finish with the soles of the feet. Put on pajamas or a warm housecoat and go back to bed.

Abdominal washing: This treatment can be done in bed before going to sleep. It is the "Kneipp sleeping pill." Move the cold, wet towel approximately twenty to forty times around your abdomen. It will help your digestion and help you fall asleep.

Frequent washings: An easy and safe way to lower a fever is a series of washings. You wash either the lower or upper extremities and repeat every fifteen minutes, six to eight times per day. The reaction you want is perspiration. Always cover the body without drying.

All washings increase the skin metabolism, help the immune system, increase circulation, provide a calming effect on the nervous system and help with rheumatic and arthritic pain. Do a washing every day, but change the body part you treat.

Water Stepping

In Europe, specially built basins along roads, in the forest, on hiking trails and in spa sanatoriums are used to collect cold water from streams or rivers. If you have hot, swollen or sweaty feet after hikes, stepping high (stork walking) through the basin until the cold water almost hurts is a wonderful, refreshing experience. Naturally, this can be done in rivers, streams or lakes, or in the bathtub! Bladder and prostate problems are contraindications.

Bath Therapy

Is the bathroom one of your favorite places? Do you think of a warm, relaxing bath after a long day's work, when stress and tension have worn you down? Do you keep several different herbal extracts handy to add to the water, depending on your mood? Herbal extracts influence your feeling of well being and a warm bath is a perfect place to relax. Bath therapy can be as simple as a bubble bath. After a warm bath have a quick cold rinse or a cold washing.

Full or partial, hot or cold, immersions in the bathtub are a big part of Kneipp Hydrotherapy. A warm bath will most likely be prescribed with the addition of an herbal extract: pine needle, meadow flowers, rosemary, balm mint, chamomile, hops, wheat bran, thyme, chestnut, lavender or others. The bath may be a half, three-quarter or full bath; a sitz bath (in a special tub that you sit in with your legs hanging out); a foot bath; or an arm bath.

An arm or foot bath might be an alternating-temperature treatment: five minutes hot, ten seconds cold, five minutes hot, ten seconds cold. It is good training for the circulatory system since it increases and decreases the diameter of the veins and arteries.

A simple cold arm bath replaces a cup of coffee; it is very uplifting and refreshing. A cold foot bath is similar to water stepping and is recommended for hot swollen legs, headaches, nose bleeds, vein and circulation problems (never with cold feet) and a nervous heart. Another form is the heat-increasing foot bath, which induces sweating to help relieve colds and flu.

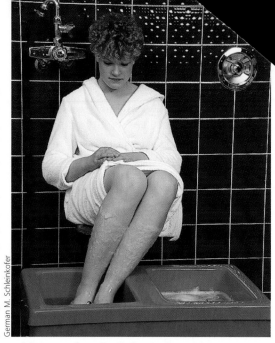

German M. Schleinkofer

An alternating-temperature foot bath is good for the circulatory system.

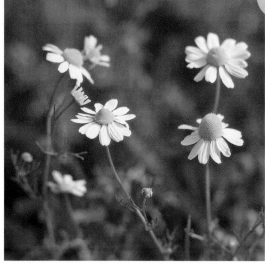

Adding chamomile to a bath will help ease inflammation, calm the nerves and treat cold and flu symptoms.

Keep the following in mind to make your bath a therapetic experience:

- Fill the bathtub first before adding the herbal extract. If you add the extract when you start the flow of water, it will produce a lot of foam you don't want. The foam forms a cool layer on the surface of the water, and also removes the protective moisture layer of the skin.
- Buy a bath thermometer for checking the temperature of the water.
- Time your bath.
- Finish a therapeutic bath with a short cool rinse from the feet up, starting on the right side. You could also have a cold, cool or temperate bath. Alternating-temperature bathing is used mainly for partial baths, such as foot or arm baths.
- You can increase the effect by either dry brushing your skin before the bath or by brushing the skin under water (see page 40). Use slow movements toward the heart and start at the right foot.
- After a therapeutic bath, half to one hour of bed rest is mandatory to achieve the full effect.
- Do not take a cold bath if your body is not totally warm!

Full, half and three-quarter baths: Fill the tub to the desired capacity with warm water (approximately 37 to 39°C (99 to 102°F). Add the herbal extract or bath oil when the tub is almost full to avoid foaming. Stir the additive into the water with either the thermometer or your arm. Step in, sit down slowly and lean back. Brushing the skin under water will increase the effectiveness of the herbal ingredients—the skin is better able to absorb the fine aromatic molecules. Remember that you also benefit through inhaling the scent of herbal bath additives. Breathing deeply and relaxing will create a great feeling of well being.

The full bath covers you up to the neck, the three-quarter bath to mid-chest level and the half bath to the waist. The choice is based on your physical condition.

A full bath is for healthy people with normal blood pressure and strong circulatory systems. Depending on length of time and the temperature, the bath will relax you or give you new energy. Twelve to fifteen minutes, certainly no more than twenty, with a temperature of 38 or 39°C (100 to 102°F) has a calming effect. Get up from the bath slowly and rinse the body with a quick, cool shower or cold washing. Start on the right foot, go up to the shoulder and down on the front of the body; repeat on the left. Rest in bed for half to one hour. Note that a warm bath in the late evening will disturb your sleep.

The three-quarter bath is similar to the full bath. The half bath is recommended as a cold immersion to increase your immune response, refresh your body, strengthen your nerves and relax you if you always feel hot and sweaty. Another form of the half bath is the temperature-increasing bath for lower-body problems. It is started with water at 33°C (91°F) and, by adding hot water over twenty minutes, the temperature is increased to 39°C (102°F). Bed rest after this one is mandatory.

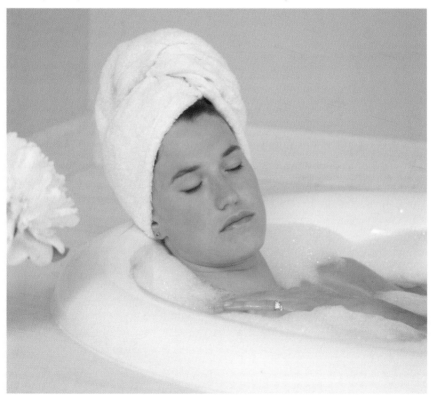

Herbal Bath Additives	Conditions Treated / Properties
Chamomile:	anti-inflammatory; calming; treats colds and flu
Pine or spruce needle:	refreshing, uplifting, energizing; treats tiredness; respiratory, circulatory and heart problems; chills; sports fatigue; muscle tension; rheumatism and arthritis
Lavender:	reduces itching and swelling of insect bites; relaxes and energizes; has a beautiful scent
Arnica:	relieves muscle aches, rheumatism and arthritic pain
Lemon balm/balm mint/melissa:	one of the most relaxing and calming herbal bath extracts; has a wonderful scent; helps you sleep; treats heart problems, migraine, rheumatism and arthritis; revitalizes sex drive
Rosemary:	improves circulation; treats heart problems; energizes—may disrupt sleep, use during daytime
Valerian:	relaxing; treats migraine, rheumatism and arthritis; helps you sleep; revitalizes sex drive
Meadow flowers/hayflowers:	calming, relaxing; smells wonderful and therefore has an effect on the respiratory system; eases muscle pain, rheumatism, arthritis, chills and migraine (place in a small porous bag, heat it and placed it on sore muscles, neck, hips or knees.)
Thyme:	coughs, bronchitis and other respiratory problems; heart problems, rheumatism and arthritis, and digestive problems
Mustard:	treats colds and flu

Foot bath: This can be a warm, cold or alternating-temperature bath, or you can use water stepping (lift each leg out of the water, to experience a change between air and water). Special foot bath tubs are available, but two garbage cans or 4-gallon paint pails will do the trick. For either, I suggest placing the containers in the bathtub; this makes for easy filling and emptying. The water has to reach up to the knee.

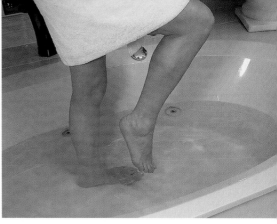

The warm foot bath, with a temperature of 37°C (99°F) for ten to fifteen minutes, promotes good sleep, helps chronic sinus problems, relieves constipation, improves circulation and builds immunity. Herbal extracts can be added. It is important to put socks on after a warm foot bath and go to bed or for a walk. Do not let your feet get cold!

The alternating-temperature foot bath requires two containers side by side: The left one is filled with warm water (38°C/100°F) and the right one with cold water. Herbal extracts can be added to the warm water. Immerse both feet in the warm water for five minutes (set your timer!), then lift the right leg out, stroke excess water off, take a deep breath, exhale and place your foot in the cold water. Follow with the left leg. Wait twenty-five seconds, lift, stroke the water off and place both legs in the warm water again. Repeat the procedure after another five minutes.

Water stepping can be done in the bathtub or in streams, rivers, lakes or the ocean.

After the last cold immersion, stroke the water off the legs, dry the soles of your feet and between the toes, and pull on long, warm socks. Go on a brisk walk or back to bed for thirty minutes. No reading, radio or television during the bed rest! Relax!

Tired, hot or swollen feet love a cold foot bath. This is also good for nosebleeds, headaches, light varicose veins, problems falling asleep, acute gout pain and even a nervous heart. Contraindications are bladder problems, very high blood pressure, sciatic inflammation and cold feet. Either fill your bathtub with cold water and "stork-walk" or use a foot bath container. Do the cold foot bath for no longer than fifteen to thirty seconds, and water stepping for about one minute. Stop when the cold "bites" you or hurts. Water stepping also can be done in streams, rivers, lakes or the ocean. It is very refreshing and energizing.

For the increasing-temperature foot bath, fill one container with lukewarm water and place your legs in the water. Dress warmly since this treatment is meant to increase the body temperature. Keep adding hot water for approximately fifteen to twenty minutes, until the bath reaches a temperature of 40°C (104°F). This may induce perspiration. Forty-five minutes to

Tired, hot or swollen feet love a cold foot bath. This is also good for nosebleeds, headaches, light varicose veins, problems falling asleep and acute gout pain.

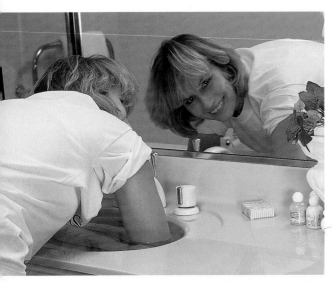

one hour of bed rest with warm covers tucked all around you is highly advisable. This is a very good way to fight an oncoming cold or flu, ease cramps and menstrual problems, and relieve headaches, chronic sinus inflammation, bladder and urinary infections and chronic cold feet. Do not use this treatment if you have varicose veins!

Arm bath: This bath can be cold or warm, or you can alternate temperatures or increase the temperature. The cold arm bath can be done in any sink, in your bathroom, in the kitchen, in a hotel–wherever you have a container or sink large enough to put your lower arms in. The water should cover the arms to a little above the elbows, but it is refreshing to just immerse your hands and arms as far as possible.

The arm bath can be done anywhere and is an excellent rejuvenator.

This treatment is better than a cup of coffee for rejuvenating yourself! I have often used it during meetings, seminars or conventions, when I got so tired that I could hardly keep my eyes open. Does your heart race or hurt without an organic reason? Is your blood pressure low and you can't fall asleep? Or is your blood pressure too high? Do you have pain after playing tennis or golf (tennis elbow)? For all these reasons, or if you just feel totally exhausted, this is the treatment for you!

Start with warm hands; stay in the cold water until you feel the cold "biting" you, approximately thirty to fifty seconds. Don't dry off, just stroke the water off and swing the arms until they are dry and warm.

For a warm arm bath, both arms should be immersed to above the elbows. An herbal extract can be added. The water temperature should be about 38°C (100°F); the length of the bath should be about twenty minutes. Sit comfortably and breathe evenly. This treatment influences the respiratory system, eases chest congestion and increases circulation in chronically cold hands. If you have suffered an angina attack, immerse only your extended left arm until help arrives.

For an arm bath of increasing temperature, start with lukewarm water and increase the temperature within twenty minutes to about 39°C (102°F). This treatment will help you recuperate after a heart attack, but make sure you don't induce perspiration. It is also good for medium-high blood pressure, headaches, asthma and head colds. Bed rest for at least half an hour is advised.

For an alternating-temperature arm bath, a double sink is needed. Special arm bath containers are available, but two rectangular plastic containers will also do. Fill one bowl or sink with warm water and the other with cold water. Herbal extracts can be added to the warm water. Place both arms in the warm water for five minutes (set the timer). Stroke the water off, take a deep breath, exhale, and immerse your arms in the cold water for fifteen to twenty seconds. Stroke the water off and repeat: five more minutes in the warm water and finish with the cold water. Do not dry, just stroke the water off and swing the arms. Go on a brisk walk or to bed for a nap.

This treatment is best done in the early afternoon. It helps to regulate blood pressure, increases circulation, and can be used for bronchitis, chronic cold hands and general tiredness. It is good training for your veins and arteries; warm water widens veins and cold constricts them.

Body Wraps, Compresses and Packs

Full or partial wraps, either cold or warm, increase circulation and detoxify the body. Cold wraps first decrease body temperature and cause deeper breathing, a slight increase in blood pressure and better metabolism. The body will react with increased temperature after a few minutes and the opposite will happen; a nice feeling of relaxation ensues and with it an eventual decrease in pain.

Hot wraps cause similar reactions. A decrease in blood pressure because of the widening of veins and arteries helps the heart and circulatory system. Depending on the length of time wrappings are left on the body, they can decrease your temperature, increase warmth or cause perspiration. Perspiring is good for detoxification or for a fever.

Compresses and packs do not surround a body part but rather are "spot" treatments; for instance, a heart compress eases a racing heart. A pack could be done with mud, linseed or cottage cheese and applied to varicose veins or to help chronic constipation. A hot hayflower pack placed across tense shoulders or an arthritic hip or knee does wonders.

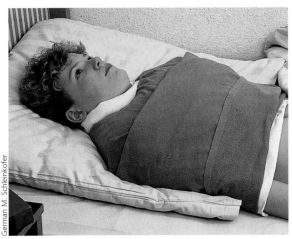

Full or partial wraps increase circulation and detoxify the body.

For wraps, compresses and packs, three pieces of material are needed: a wet, inner part that is placed on the skin, a middle part covering the wet layer and an outer layer to keep cold air from getting in and warmth from getting out. The middle layer should be a little larger than the outer layer so that you will not have to wash the outer layer every time you use it. Additions such as vinegar, salt or herbal extracts increase the effectiveness of the wraps. For home use I recommend sticking to the partial wraps; whole-body wraps are best left to professionals. To make your wrap you need three pieces of material:

- an inner wrapper of rough cotton or linen to absorb water well and retain cold or heat
- a middle layer of thicker cotton of a finer weave and slightly larger than the inner layer to protect against leakage
- an outer layer of wool or flannel to retain warmth

The size of the wrapper depends on the body part to be treated. You can cut up old blankets, or use kitchen towels or baby blankets, or you can buy the materials you need. Ready-made wrappers are available, made out of the right materials in various sizes.

Wrapping can be done with cold water or warm/hot water, with or without herbal additives. Wrapping goes all around the body or body part. When doing a "pack," instead of wrapping the inner layer, fold it, dip it in water and place it on the part being treated (for example, the liver, abdomen or stomach), then wrap the middle layer around, followed by the wool or flannel outer cloth. No air should be able to get to the inner, wet part, so the middle and outer cloths have to be tightly wrapped. Wrapping is done in bed. No reading, radio, TV or conversation, please! Your whole body has to be tucked under the covers.

The wrapper stays on until it changes temperature; that is, until a cold one gets warm or a warm one gets cold, approximately forty-five minutes to an hour. After removal, another ten minutes in a warm bed are beneficial. A wrap of either temperature will increase the warmth of the body, help to relax muscle tension, decrease pain and have a positive effect on blood pressure and the heart. If for some reason the body does not respond to a cold wrap with increasing warmth after about five minutes but feels cold or chilly, the wrap must be removed. The body has to be warm before and after the wrap is placed.

Lower-leg wrap: A cold wrap is usually used. The wet inner part is tightly wrapped around the calf, followed by the middle and outer layers. The wrapper stays on for twenty to thirty minutes. It feels wonderful after long hikes, after you've been on your feet all day and if you have sunburn, high blood pressure, inflammation, vein pain, general nervousness or problems falling asleep. Do not use this treatment if you are chilled to the bone or have the flu or a urinary tract infection.

This treatment is the "Aspirin" of Kneipp Hydrotherapy; it helps reduce fever! For this treatment the cold wrapper is removed as soon as it feels warm; repeat three or four times. Perform the treatment several times throughout the day if necessary.

A hot hayflower pack placed across tense shoulders, or an arthritic hip or knee, does wonders.

Wet Socks
Instead of the lower- or full-leg wrap, you can use wet socks. This is a simple treatment for varicose veins, irritability and insomnia. Two pairs of knee-high socks are needed. The inner ones should be linen or rough cotton, which hold the cold water nicely; pull a pair of warm, soft woolen socks over the wet ones. For sleep problems you can leave the socks on all night or pull them off when they wake you up. For varicose veins they should come off before they get warm. Never use cold wet socks if you have cold feet or an acute bladder infection.

Cold abdominal wrap: Cover the area between the waist and legs. This can be done with an all-around inner wrapper or by folding it and placing it on the abdomen. The middle layer is quickly wrapped around, followed by the outer cover, which could be a large towel or blanket. If this wrap does not warm the area within six to ten minutes, place a hot-water bottle on top or remove the wrap.

Problems such as constipation, gas, stomach upset and high blood pressure can be treated. Menstruation and urinary infections are contraindications.

Cold or hot chest wrap: The wrappers need to be wide enough to cover the chest between the underarms and waist, and your body has to be warm. Leave the wrap on for forty-five to seventy-five minutes until the chest feels comfortably warm. The cold wrap is recommended for acute bronchitis, pneumonia and other chest inflammations. It helps to dilute bronchial fluids, lowers fever, decreases pain and increases circulation in the chest area. Bed rest is mandatory.

The warm chest wrap is recommended for chronic bronchitis and mucus removal. You can rub the chest with aromatic oils such as wintergreen, menthol or tea tree oil before the wrapper is placed.

Cold neck wrap: For the neck wrap, you can use a long linen towel folded lengthwise to be just as wide as the neck. Dip one end of the towel in cold water, press out the excess and wrap around the neck so that the dry part is on top. Secure with safety pins. For acute conditions remove the wrap as soon as it no longer feels cold.

Sore throats, hyperthyroidism and chronic or acute sinus problems will respond to this treatment. For chronic problems repeat nightly for several weeks and leave it on overnight. Should a sore throat or other pain increase, remove the wrap immediately.

The cold neck wrap is useful when treating a sore throat, hyperthyroidism and sinus problems.

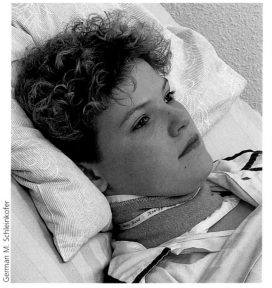

German M. Schleinkofer

Hot pack: In Kneipp Hydrotherapy, meadow or hay flowers are used in a linen bag, steamed and applied hot to a sore shoulder, knee, hip or stomach, with the area then wrapped as usual. The duration of the treatment is forty-five minutes. In lieu of meadow flowers you can use hot mashed potatoes (no lumps, please!), a hot-water bottle or a heated gel pack.

Cold pack: To ease varicose veins, cottage cheese, loam or healing earth is applied to a piece of gauze and placed on the area, wrapped and left for forty-five minutes to an hour. Loam and healing earth remove skin moisture, so rub cream or lotion into the skin after the treatment.

Cold heart compress: Fold one of your inner-layer pieces to size, dip it in cold water, remove the excess and place on the heart and wrap like a chest wrap. This helps to calm a racing, nervous heart.

Help! Which Treatment for Which Problem?

Kneipp Hydrotherapy at home is for the prevention and stabilization of a wide range of conditions. It is energizing and provides life enhancement. After you have been ill, your health will return more quickly with hydrotherapy. It helps to improve your immune system. You become stronger and more resistant. But remember that Kneipp Hydrotherapy is by no means a replacement for medical attention and treatment; use it as a complementary method of health care, and tell your health-care provider that you are using it.

Cold Hands and Feet

This is a common problem caused by poor circulation; it can also be inherited. Ailments such as low blood pressure, diabetes and hypothyroidism cause circulation problems. Exercise and movement is important. Do not sit still for long periods of time. Seniors tend to suffer from poor circulation if they lead a sedentary lifestyle. Certain medications, such as the contraceptive pill and hypertension drugs, can be the cause.

Kneipp Hydrotherapy uses dry brushing, the warm arm bath, the alternating-temperature arm bath, the warm or alternating-temperature foot bath and the alternating-temperature arm and knee rinses to improve the condition.

Kneipp Hydrotherapy at home is for the prevention and stabilization of a wide range of conditions; it is energizing and provides life enhancement.

Heart Problems

Exercise and hydrotherapy strengthen the heart and circulatory system.

Circulatory problems can lead to heart disease. A sedentary lifestyle, improper diet and lack of exercise are contributors. Heart palpitations, irregular heartbeat, a racing heart, stabbing pain, anxiety and panic attacks are early warning signs. If a professional diagnosis does not reveal any organic causes for your discomfort, it is most likely related to nervous stress, tension and unresolved psychological problems.

Over a period of a year, daily monitoring of blood pressure after walking, jogging, swimming, table tennis and dancing has taught me that during exercise the pulse rate goes up but the pressure goes down. Watching television, reading, sitting at a computer or chatting on the phone has shown me that this type of activity brings the pulse rate down, but the blood pressure up.

These observations proved to me that exercise and hydrotherapy strengthen the heart and circulatory system. During one year I was able to reduce my hypertension medication to half and during the active summer months I did not need it at all.

My doctor, who was both surprised and happy, said, "You've proven it can be done, with determination and discipline!" So be active! And remember: Kneipp Hydrotherapy is used as complementary therapy and does not replace medical treatment!

I recommend dry brushing in the morning before the bath or shower, alternating-temperature arm and knee rinses, alternating-temperature arm and foot baths and the warm three-quarter bath. You can do cold water stepping or brief cold immersions of the feet if they are warm. A cold arm bath, for both or for just the extended left arm, of fifteen to twenty seconds' duration will help to tone and strengthen the heart and is also useful for acute angina attacks or pain radiating from the chest down into the left arm. If necessary, put the patient at rest and apply a cold wrapper around the extended left arm until the ambulance arrives.

Headaches and Migraine

Women are especially prone to headaches, particularly during or just prior to menstruation. Muscle tension in the upper back and shoulders from prolonged sitting, poor posture, eye strain and loud noise also can cause headaches. A shortage of oxygen in an overheated room, food allergies, changes in blood pressure and low blood sugar are other causes.

Kneipp Hydrotherapy uses cold immersions of the feet (if your feet are warm), alternating-temperature foot baths, alternating-temperature knee or hip rinses and often a cold arm bath. A hot compress to the neck might be helpful for a tension headache.

Migraines are often disabling. Sometimes one-sided, they can cause vomiting and nausea, sore eyes, muscle tension, a dull pain in the forehead or back of the head or a piercing pain in the temples. Just taking a pain killer does not solve the problem. Migraines affect the blood vessels of the brain. Since these can be trained like muscles, regular Kneipp treatments with alternating warm and cold water over a long period of time offer help.

Heat dilates the blood vessels and cold constricts them. Through foot and leg treatments, the reflex arc, the nerve path from the point of origin (feet) to the nerve center (head) influences the vessels all over the body. The result is better circulation in the head and brain.

Kneipp Hydrotherapy suggests alternating-temperature showers, alternating-temperature leg and arm rinses and baths, a three-quarter bath at 38°C (100°F) for twenty minutes with a cold finish and cold water stepping in the bathtub. At the onset of a migraine a temperature-increasing foot bath may be of help to avert it, or to at least help avoid the worst of it.

Colds and Flu

To avoid colds and flu, improve your immune system during the warm season. Make sure your feet are never cold since this lowers resistance. Observe strict hygiene, wash your hands, clean doorknobs, etc. during cold season and avoid crowds.

Influenza viruses are stronger and more infectious than cold bugs. While a cold might be accompanied by a slight rise in body temperature, the flu can cause a high fever, total exhaustion and aches all over the body. A sore throat, dry cough, runny nose and a severe headache can be part of the package. Left

Kneipp Hydrotherapy uses hot, sweat-inducing baths or wraps to treat colds and flu.

untreated, the flu can develop into pneumonia, which can be fatal for older or weaker people.

Kneipp Hydrotherapy uses hot, sweat-inducing baths or wraps to treat colds and flu. Use a three-quarter or full bath if you have a strong heart, the half bath and temperature-increasing foot bath or cold chest wraps if you are weaker. Bed rest after these baths is mandatory. Inhaling steam from water boiled with chamomile, and drinking Linden tea, also helps.

Fever

The body raises its temperature to combat bacteria and viruses, which do not thrive in an environment with a temperature over 39°C (102°F). It is therefore not always wise to reduce a fever. Exceptions are fevers higher than this, the "burning-up" sensation in older pneumonia patients and high fevers in very young children. It is important to avoid dehydration through perspiration. Drinking lots of liquids is important.

Kneipp Hydrotherapy can induce a fever with hot or temperature-increasing three-quarter or full baths, a temperature-increasing foot bath and heavy, total snug coverage of the body in bed. To reduce a fever, a cold wrapper around both calves is used. It stays on until it gets warm (twenty minutes) and might be repeated several times. Take your temperature between treatments; the fever should go down gradually.

Rheumatism and Arthritis

The "morphine of the Kneipp Cure," the hayflower pack, is absolute king in providing relief.

Symptoms of rheumatism and arthritis can appear at any age. More than one hundred different forms of arthritis are known, but the most common are rheumatoid arthritis and osteoarthritis. Osteoarthritis is an inflammation of the joints. There can be pain-free periods with this condition, but in time the joint wears down and the pain can be constant and crippling.

Rheumatoid arthritis is worse. This inflammation can cause deformation at an early age. Fingers and toes are often affected first, but wrists, knees, spine and ankles are endangered as well. The pain can wander through the body from joint to joint, and attacks can come on suddenly.

Eating nonacidic food is very important to keeping the condition at bay; in fact, a total change of lifestyle is often necessary. Kneipp Hydrotherapy suggests washings, wraps and rinses.

When an inflammation is present, the colder the treatment, the better, even to the point of using ice packs or rubbing ice on the skin. Some individuals find more relief with warm treatments. In that case, alternating-temperature foot and arm baths are suggested. The "morphine of the Kneipp Cure," the hayflower pack, is absolute king in providing relief. Other additives could include cottage cheese on a gauze cloth for a wrap.

Digestive Problems

Constipation is a widespread problem. Refined food, lack of fiber, stress, nervousness, not enough liquids, lack of exercise and disorder in your daily activities are some of the reasons. Take time when the urge appears! Elimination should occur once a day or more often.

Laxatives are no solution since they increase the muscle weakness of the intestines and colon. If food waste is kept too long in the body, other problems and diseases will occur. Bad breath, skin eruptions and headaches are only the simpler ones.

Several conventional medications are contributing factors; diuretics, iron preparations, antacids, antidepressants and pain killers are among them. An under-active thyroid gland also can be a cause. People in the western world experience waste holding of up to 36 hours and more, which leads to toxicity in the blood stream. In the eastern world, up to 18 hours is the norm. As Father Kneipp said, "Death sits in the colon!"

Kneipp Hydrotherapy recommends cold abdominal wraps. Vinegar can be added to the water. Other treatments include circular washings with cold water and vinegar on the abdomen. Move a folded linen cloth, dipped in the liquid and slightly pressed out, in a circular motion clockwise around the abdomen thirty to forty times, rewetting the cloth when it feels warm. This can be done in bed in the early morning.

Stay in bed for another

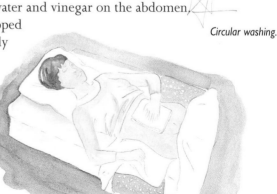

Circular washing.

half an hour after the treatment or until the urge to go to the washroom makes you get up. You can also use a warm or cold sitz bath (in lieu of a sitz bath, use the half bath). Additives to the cold water could include vinegar or salt.

Insomnia

A lukewarm half bath will help you fall asleep.

Always go to bed at the same time. Do not watch an exciting movie or read an interesting book prior to sleep. Try to relax and mentally prepare for the bedroom, which should be for sleeping and lovemaking only. A lukewarm (less than 38°C/100°F) half bath for about eight minutes will help you fall asleep. Dry only between your legs and between your toes; elsewhere, just stroke the water off, put pajamas on and go straight to bed.

A cold wrap around the lower body is effective, as is a lower-body cold washing without drying. If your feet are warm, you can use wet socks. Water stepping for twenty seconds in a bathtub full of cold water is helpful. If you have a problem sleeping throughout the night, try doing another cold lower-body washing. If that fails, perform an alternating-temperature knee or hip rinse.

Sexual Dysfunction

Impotence in men and a low sex drive in women have many causes in addition to hormonal changes. Fatigue, depression, no time or opportunity, lack of trust in the partner, drugs for depression or high blood pressure, coffee, alcohol, smoking, street drugs, an improper diet and mineral deficiencies can all contribute. Hormonal changes can cause vaginal dryness, which might cause pain for both partners. Mental attitude and strong emotions such as anger, anxiety and guilt can decrease the sex drive, while declarations of love and desire will improve it. Age is no reason to lose interest in sex, since the need for emotional closeness remains. An 89-year-old woman said to me, "It changes alright, but it never stops."

Kneipp Hydrotherapy recommends dry brushing (preferably done by the partner), cold half baths, cold lower-body washings, alternating-temperature sitz baths and warm three-quarter baths. It is said that three to four weeks of Kneipp therapy in a controlled setting will turn a monogamous person towards polygamy if the partner is not around!

The Five Pillars of the Kneipp System . . . . .

Father Kneipp insisted that the human body had to be treated as a whole. You can't just treat a symptom; you must look at the whole body for true healing to take place. Healing is not simply giving the patient a pain killer; the reason for the pain has to be found and treated. Kneipp said, "I have found that no true healing takes place if body, mind and spirit are not united." He often saw the true reason for health problems as what we today would describe as stress. It all starts in the mind. Inner conflicts and unhappiness cause dis-ease. Dis-ease is the beginning of disease.

> **Burnout and Stress**
> The Kneipp Five Pillar System is the best remedy for whatever stresses plague you. It increases immune response and circulation, it stabilizes and strengthens, and it relaxes and energizes. Making Kneipp's water therapy part of your daily life routine pays great dividends. You will feel and look younger as the years go by.

His own success in returning to health by using water was multiplied by the thousands of people who sought him out. As a boy, accompanying his mother collecting herbs for tea and medicine, he learned that God grew a plant for every ill. "Every animal knows what to look for when it is sick; humans have lost the ability." Kneipp was one of the first to collect and catalog herbs.

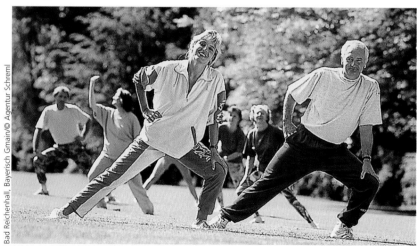

Bad Reichenhall, Bayerisch Gmain/© Agentur Schreml

Another of Kneipp's insights was the value of exercise. He directed patients to chop wood before or after the water treatments he administered. King, bishop or farmer, everybody was treated equally. He condemned refined food and recommended simple bread, grains, vegetables and raw milk (unlike the commercial, pasteurized milk we are offered in the stores today). He also maintained that people who couldn't tolerate beer made from wheat once in a while must be very ill!

As the Father Confessor for a convent, he urged the nuns to work in the garden and fields saying, "Work is a form of prayer." His philosophy eventually became known as the "Five Pillar System," and is based on these principles:

- water therapy
- nature's apothecary
- he who rests, rusts
- let thy food be thy medicine
- pray and work

We have already discussed Kneipp's first pillar, water therapy, in detail. Let's take a look at the others.

Nature's Apothecary

Kneipp said, "God let the plants and herbs grow for our benefit: We should learn to know and use them to prevent, ease and cure our ills. With every step we take in nature, we will see new

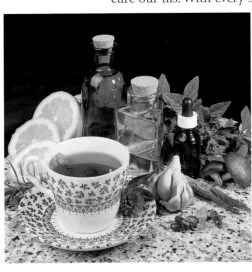

plants of great advantage in the healing arts. For many years I used herbs in my cure with the greatest success."

Through industrialization and advances in science, chemistry and technology, a new wave of incredible, effective medical developments took place. Incurable diseases were brought under control and folkloric medicine (including herbal treatments) was forgotten. But lately, fueled by an unprecedented increase in new, unknown and drug-resistant viruses and bacteria, a trend toward the use of natural remedies is gaining momentum. Father Kneipp's basic belief that an ounce of pre-vention is worth a pound of cure is the cry of the day. The scientific community has created a trustworthy base for "folk" medicine–objective research and controlled studies are the foundation of modern phytotherapy, or plant medicine.

He Who Rests, Rusts

Industrial developments, an eight-hour work day and previously unheard of free time brought our modern day an increase in participation in sports and travel to foreign countries. In Father Kneipp's time, exercise as such was unknown. Health seekers who came from all over the continent for his advice, poor or rich, were required to chop wood to warm up or stay warm. The nuns in his charge were told in no uncertain terms that praying alone made them weak and that work was a form of prayer. Milking cows, shovel-ing manure and working in fields and gardens was soon part of their days in the convent. To work, move and walk barefoot through the grassy pastures became part of the cure and remains so today.

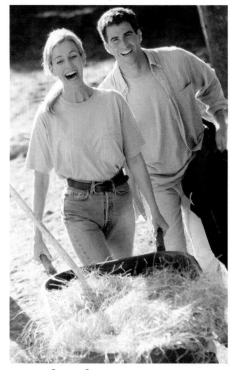

Sports and exercise are filling a large part of our free time and we know that they increase our quality of life and extend our life span. Father Kneipp said if we walked more, everything would be better! In his time, more than one hundred years ago, the order of the day was walking; only the wealthy had horses, wagons and carriages. Physical work, such as chopping wood to warm up your body before, and keep it warm after one of his treatments, was a big part of his system.

Today, we see an unprecedented increase in body awareness and we know how important exercise and movement are. It seems like everybody is into it. Exercise and movement keep all the parts of the body functioning through improved oxygen supply via increased circulation. Kneipp warned us that disease can begin in the blood. If we can clean up the blood, we can prevent and cure disease.

If you don't think you have time for an exercise class, walk everywhere. Walk up the stairs, even if you don't make all of them. Turn all your daily work into exercises: stretch when you reach into your cupboard, bend over when you make your bed. Work both sides of the body when you vacuum, wash your car and your windows, even if it takes longer. Walk back and forth in your house often, get up during all commercials if you watch TV and do something else. Get a bike to go to work. Don't sit for extended periods at a desk. You've heard the phrase "use it or lose it." Use your body!

Dry brushing: As mentioned at the beginning of this book, I learned about the Kneipp System because of my poor circulation. The attending physician in the Kneipp sanatorium I was sent to "confiscated" my conventional medications and gave me my first lesson in dry brushing. With a rough sisal mitt and back-strap, I had to brush my whole body every morning until the skin was rosy pink. Often I brushed before the bath

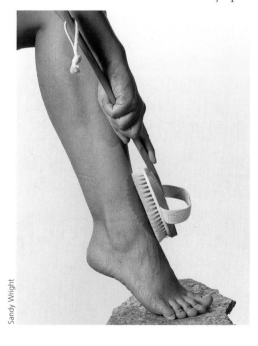

Sandy Wright

treatments to enable the skin to absorb the herbal additives better. When my feet were cold I brushed my legs. Now, more than forty years later, I am still brushing! A positive side effect is the health of the skin tissue, tighter breasts, no flab on the abdomen and no scaly skin anywhere.

I consider dry brushing the most important passive exercise. It can be done sitting or standing, and it takes only five minutes. It is better than a cup of coffee to get you going. Husband and wife can do it to each other, but watch out! It is invigorating and stimulating; you might not get to work on time! Do the dry brushing daily before your shower.

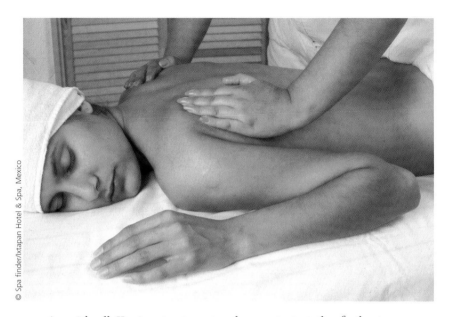

As with all Kneipp treatments, always start at the farthest spot from the heart: The right foot. You redirect the blood flow away from the heart, easing its work. Brush the right foot and leg up to the torso until the skin is flushed. Brush the left foot and leg until you have the same effect. Brush your abdomen, starting at the appendix site, and move up and around the belly button. To achieve high color here takes a little longer. Brush your right arm, starting with the hand and moving up to and including the shoulder; repeat on the left side. Brush across the chest, but be careful not to brush your nipples. Move around the breasts in a figure eight motion; don't press too hard, you are dealing with more sensitive tissue. Brush the chest until you see the increase in circulation.

Massage

Body massage, full or partial, is another form of passive exercise. A weekly massage would be a dream; it not only relaxes the muscles and eases tension, it helps to remove toxins, it is stimulating, tones the nerves, is an antidepressant and helps to eliminate pain. Don't worry if it hurts a bit; sometimes the massage therapist has to go into the deeper layers to do a good job. Acupressure, shiatsu, nerve point massage and reflexology are all beneficial if other, active exercise for some reason is limited or impossible.

Women with pendulous breasts should hold them in their other hand when brushing and be careful not to scratch the skin with the brush. Do not brush the front of your neck or your face. Brush your backside starting under the buttocks. Go around them, then brush up the middle of your back up to the neck. For the back I recommend a knitted sisal or horse hair back-strap. It has handles on both ends and you can pull it back and forth with the pressure you like. Pulling it across the back of your neck also eliminates a lot of muscle tension after a strenuous tense day.

Let Thy Food Be Thy Medicine

Hippocrates, the Greek physician who lived from 460 to 377 BC, and known as the Father of Medicine, knew and preached the value of food. Kneipp believed in neither over- nor under-eating, and was the one who taught us that our food should be our medicine. Father Kneipp promoted freshly milled simple grains, lots of vegetables and fruit, nothing overcooked, meat only occasionally, clean fresh water and herbal tea and, once in while, a glass of wine or wheat beer.

Hundreds of people gathered every day to hear Father Kneipp speak about lifestyle choices. One of the topics he often discussed was food and drink. Since he promoted simple peasant food such as bread, soup, cottage cheese, fruit and vegetables, he steamed about excesses: "All of you want to eat like pigs, but nobody wants to die!" He also said, "When you feel you have eaten, you have already eaten too much."

> **Kneipp on Lifestyle Choices**
> Shoes were another topic Kneipp groaned about when speaking to people about their choices. He endorsed the sandal as a way to provide air and sunshine for the feet. "How can your pair of feet carry you through life without complaint if you keep them imprisoned?" One could say that Kneipp was ahead of his time, since his ideas sound pretty modern! What he said at the end of the 19th century is valid today as we start the 21st century.

Doesn't all this sound familiar? Have we reverted to 19th century teachings? Or was Kneipp ahead of his time? Don't scientists tell us we should eat broccoli to prevent cancer, carrots and melon to improve our brittle bones, fish to build better

cells, some meat to replace lost iron and vitamin C to counter-
act the lack of it in unripe fruit? And what about all the other
antioxidants needed to help the body deal with poisons in the
environment? The list is endless.

Simple and healthy meals: Father Kneipp was raised as a very
poor boy. He learned early to appreciate having food at all. When
he was seven years old, he reached for the salt to have with his
potatoes. His mother was quick to slap his face and tell him,
"You have not earned your salt yet."

Father Kneipp felt food should be pure, mostly vegetarian,
not overcooked and not too plentiful. Hearty bread, fruit, vegetables, cottage cheese and simple soups are what he grew up
on. Only on high holidays and maybe on Sunday was meat
served. I remember that during the week only my father ate
meat. Kneipp said, "When you feel you have eaten, you have
already eaten too much!"

Many people reward themselves and their children with
food. "If you eat your meal, you will get dessert." "If you do
your home work, I'll give you a chocolate bar." "Why shouldn't
I eat, what else do I have?"

Today's trend is toward a healthy, balanced
lifestyle. Food is a large part of it. The new cook-
books reflect this. Every magazine or newspaper
recipe section features "modern" recipes. Our
biggest problem is the toxicity of all our food,
caused by radiation, pesticides, and loss of
enzymes, vitamins and minerals. Lack of crop
rotation allows insects to breed. Crops are
grown on the same parcel of land with the help
of fertilizers, long after all nutrients have been
leached out of the soil. One of our staple foods,
the potato, is an example. The trace mineral
selenium, necessary for a healthy potato (and
our equilibrium) is barely present in most of
the soil in North America today.

Do you remember the taste of a tomato or
carrot grown in your back yard? And how they
smelled? I do. I cannot find a tomato or carrot
like that, not even in the organic food shops,

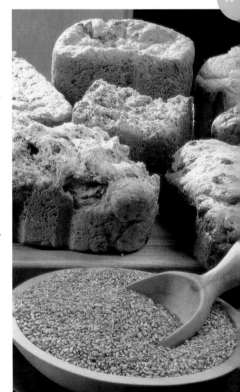

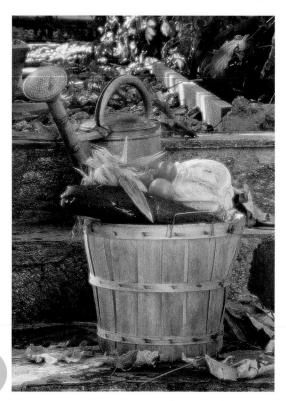

though shopping for organic food has become ever more important. It is no longer just the spraying that is the problem; the degeneration, manipulation and genetic changes are serious health threats.

We cannot even choose if we do not want to eat the "new" generation of food, because there is no information on the products. Be aware! To return the land to a balanced state after years of abuse takes several years, but more and more farmers are making the attempt. If you have a chance, plant a garden and grow some of your own food.

The freshest food is always the healthiest food. Eat lots of salads, fruits and steamed vegetables. Avoid refined flour, sugar and salt; all canned or packaged goods; and ready-made dinners. When shopping, avoid the center aisles of the grocery store. All the healthier stuff is around the outside: fruit and vegetables, milk and cheese, fresh meat and fish. Don't even look at all the sweets at the checkout counter!

To be slim and trim eat about half of what you think you need because you don't need it, you just want it. Why do you think there are so many successful weight clinics? Do you have power over your body or do you need a crutch? Let thy food be thy medicine!

Ora et Labora (Pray and Work)

The Latin phrase *Ora et Labora* really expresses what Kneipp believed life is all about. Just as he told the nuns in Bavaria, it is not enough to just pray; you have to work. Work makes the body stronger, and if God gave you a body, He also expects you to take care of it. You cannot do that by being a "couch potato." "A healthy mind lives in a healthy body!"

The stress surrounding us has caused a trend toward the spiritual, to find our center, to rest our soul, to seek and find God, to meditate and to pray. Father Kneipp said that he had never seen healing take place until the mind was at peace with God. Kneipp called this "the order in life." It is the final pillar on which the Kneipp System rests.

Order and balance in your life: As a priest and confessor, Kneipp observed first hand that inner problems made people sick. Emotional problems affect your mental ability to deal with those same problems; mental uneasiness causes stress and tension, tension causes changes in the nervous system, the nervous system affects the hormonal system, and this affects all the other body systems. Faith can help ease the load if you truly believe. Father Kneipp preached order, which for him meant cleaning up your act and living according to the Bible and the Ten Commandments. Every religion teaches principles of honor and, if followed, there is order in the mind. The mind overrides physical limitations. "How the man thinketh, so is he." Or listen to Hamlet: "Nothing is good or bad, but thinking makes it so."

Kneipp also talked of balance, balance between working and resting, eating and fasting, feasting and meditating. Balance in all phases of life. Kneipp was a beekeeper, and working with his bees helped him find his center. We need a hobby or something that allows us to step out of ourselves and to just "be," to feel balanced, centered. To feel well. We cannot achieve total wellness without order and balance in our lives. We have to feel connected to a higher being, to the universe, to something! Call it what you will; we need a spiritual life.

Order in life also means organizing your day. Get up at the same time; go to bed at the same time. Eat at the same time; eliminate at the same time. Exceptions should not become the rule. Sit down and take time for eating, and chew your food well. If conversing over a meal, keep it light and easy. Have a sense of direction in your life; do not drift like a leaf in the river.

Act according to your standards and values. Take time for your health. Father Kneipp warns, "He who has no time to care for his health daily will have to have time when he is sick for weeks and months, and will finally be seriously ill."

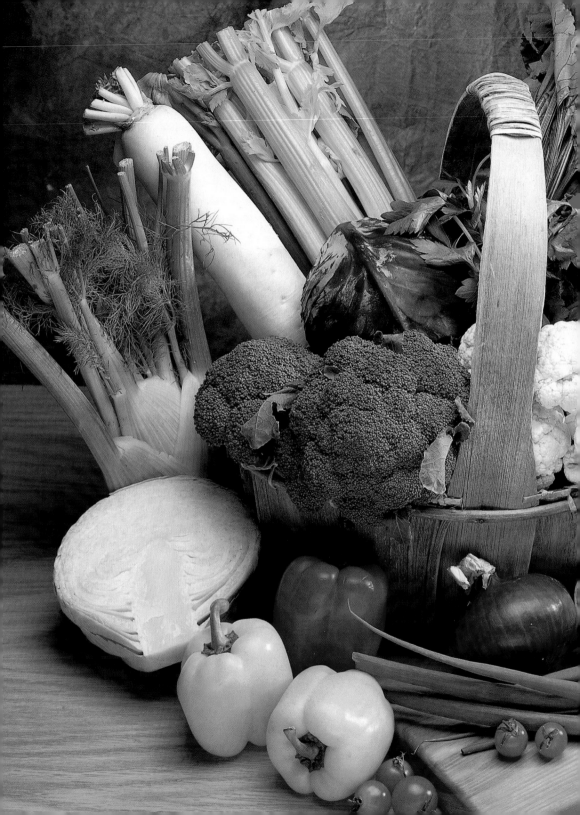

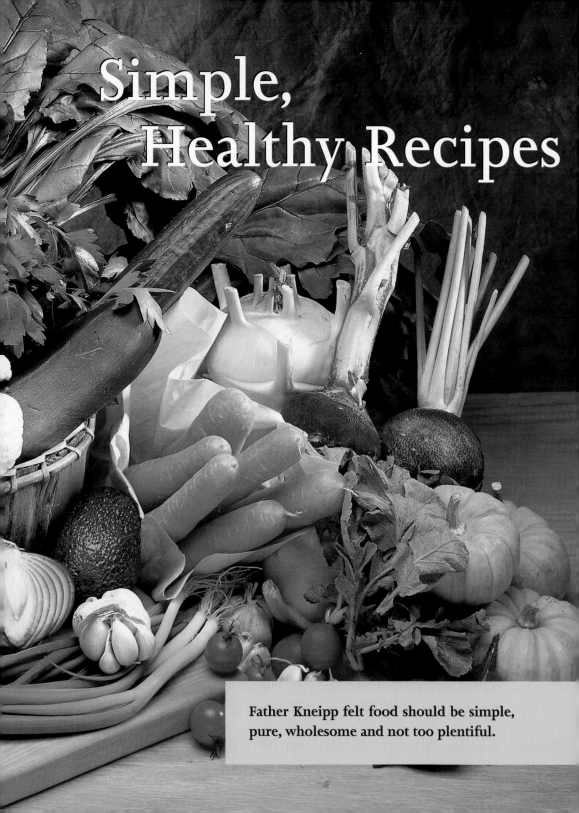

Simple,
Healthy Recipes

Father Kneipp felt food should be simple,
pure, wholesome and not too plentiful.

Papaya and Grapefruit with Kamut

Father Kneipp advocated eating whole grains. He would have loved the wonderfully healthful Kamut flakes that we can easily buy from our health food store today.

½ **papaya**

½ **grapefruit**

I **cup (150 g) unsweetened Kamut flakes**

½ **cup (125 ml) freshly squeezed orange juice**

Cut the papaya into 1/2" (1 cm) cubes (after removing the skin and seeds). Peel and segment the grapefruit. In a large bowl, thoroughly combine the fruit, Kamut and juice. Serve immediately.

Serves 1

Millet Puffs with Fruit

Any healthy cereal is an exciting and tasty treat when fresh fruit is added.

¼ **cup (100 g) fresh strawberries**

¼ **cup (120 g) fresh papaya, cut in ½" (1 cm) cubes**

½ **banana, sliced**

¼ **cup (120 g) fresh grapefruit segments**

½ **cup (120 g) millet puffs**

I **tbsp pure maple syrup**

In a bowl, thoroughly combine the fresh fruit and millet puffs. Drizzle maple syrup over top and serve immediately.

Serves 1

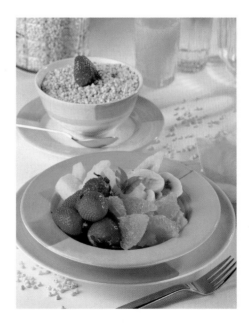

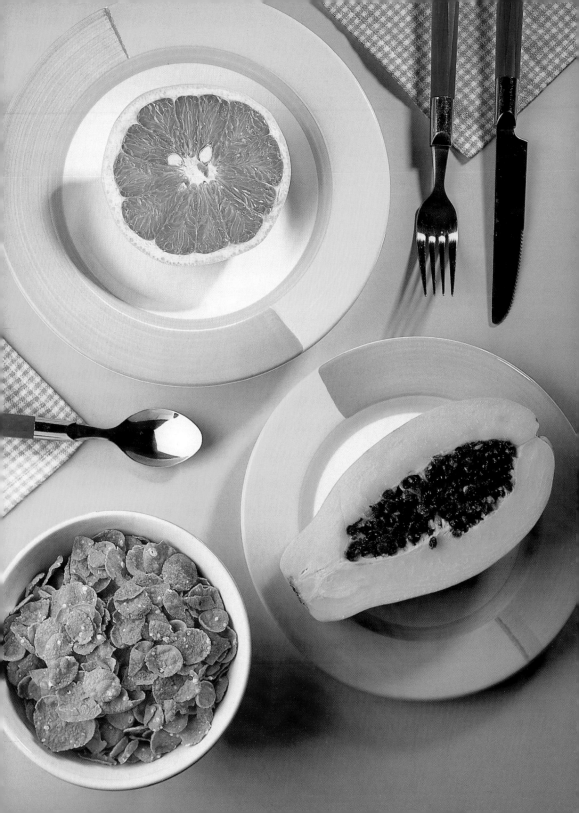

Spinach and Strawberry Salad

Do you know why Popeye is a symbol of strength whenever he eats spinach? Because spinach, especially when eaten raw, provides strength through its many valuable nutrients and high iron content. Along with the vitamin C in strawberries, this salad combination is bursting with nutrition.

4 cups (1 lb or 450 g)
baby leaf spinach

2 cups (240 g) **fresh
strawberries, hulled and
quartered**

2 cups (240 g) **teardrop or
cherry tomatoes**

½ cup (100 g) **roasted
sliced almonds**

**Sea salt and freshly
ground pepper to taste**

Dressing:

½ cup (120 ml) **cold-
pressed almond oil**

**2 tbsp freshly squeezed
lemon or lime juice**

**2 tbsp unsweetened
strawberry jam**

**1 tbsp fresh tarragon,
chopped**

Toss all ingredients, except for the almonds. Mix dressing ingredients, pour over salad and toss again. Divide into serving bowls, season and sprinkle with almonds.

Serves 2

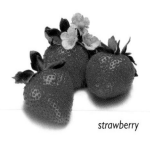

strawberry

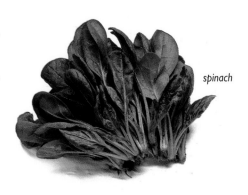

spinach

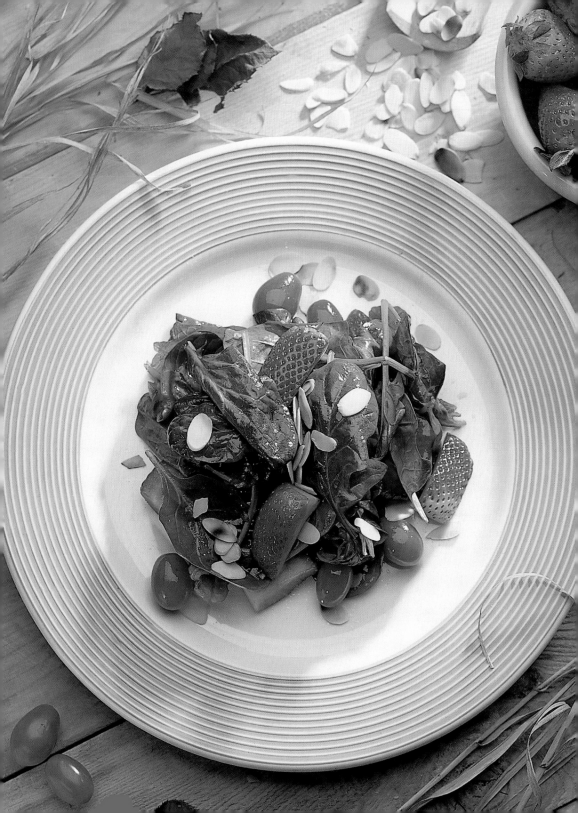

Squash Soup with Garlic Croutons

Father Kneipp encouraged people to eat simple soups as he did when he was growing up. Vegetables, spices and healthy broth add up to a wonderfully healthful meal in a bowl. The tasty croutons are not like the cubed type we're used to buying in a box. These croutons are served as whole slices. They are wonderful in the soup–a crispy contrast to this delicious, smooth dish.

1 large butternut squash

2 tbsp extra-virgin olive oil

1 cup (240 g) celery, diced

1 cup (240 g) onion, diced

1 cup (240 g) carrots, diced

3 cloves garlic, minced

1 qt (1 L) vegetable stock or water

Pinch ground cloves, coriander and ground nutmeg

2 sage leaves

Sea salt and freshly ground pepper to taste

2 tbsp organic butter

Fresh cilantro or parsley for garnish

Garlic Croutons:

4 slices dark rye bread

1 clove garlic, halved

2 tbsp extra-virgin olive oil

In a large pot, heat the oil on medium heat, add all the vegetables and the garlic and sauté until translucent. Add vegetable stock, cover and simmer over medium heat for 5 minutes.

Add spices and sage and cook for another 5 to 7 minutes until all the vegetables are tender. Season with salt and pepper.

Place the soup in a blender and blend until smooth. Return soup to the pot and add butter, simmering on low heat for 5 minutes.

To prepare the croutons brush the bread slices with olive oil and bake in the oven at 380°F (200°C) or in a frying pan, turning once, until both sides are golden brown. Remove from heat and rub both sides of the bread with the garlic clove.

Place the croutons in the soup, garnish with cilantro and serve immediately.

Serves 4

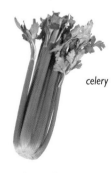

celery

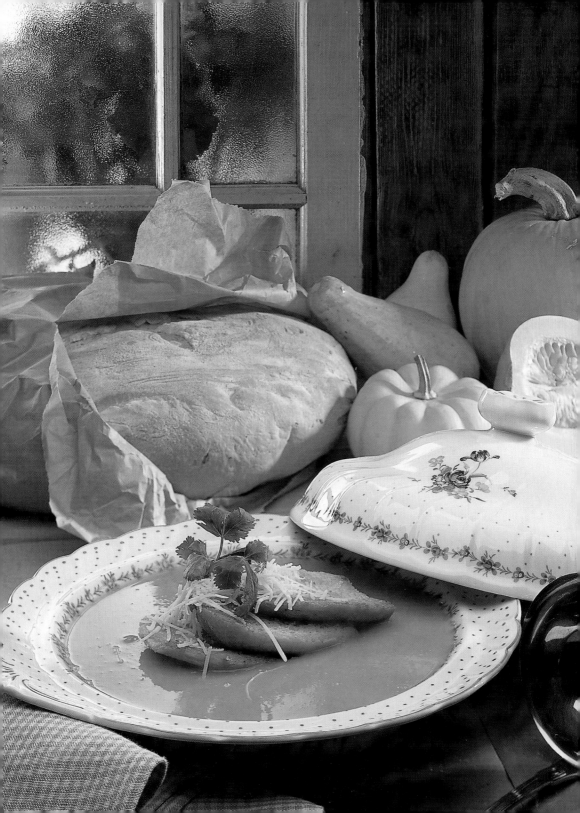

Supa de Verde

The Italians claim to have invented this soup, however, the Spanish contradict them by claiming it as their own. In the end it doesn't matter who first stirred this soup, it is so tasty and healthy both should get an award for inventing it, in my opinion.

3 tbsp extra-virgin
    olive oil

½ lb (225 g) **celery, cut in
    1" long pieces**

½ lb (225 g) **leeks, cut in
    ½" slices**

1 ½ qt (1 ½ l) **vegetable
    stock or water**

2 tbsp apple cider

5 cloves garlic, minced

3 bay leaves

2 sprigs fresh rosemary

½ lb (225 g) **Brussels
    sprouts, trimmed and
    halved**

½ lb (225 g) **asparagus
    spears**

½ lb (225 g) **broccoli
    florets**

½ lb (225 g) **green string
    beans, trimmed and
    halved**

½ lb (225 g) **zucchini, cut in
    1" diagonals**

1 white onion, chopped

**Sea salt and freshly ground pepper
    to taste**

2 tbsp butter (optional)

In a large pot, heat the oil over medium heat; add celery and leeks and sauté for 2 to 3 minutes. Add the vegetable stock, cider, herbs and remaining vegetables. Season with salt and pepper. Cover, bring to a boil and then simmer for 10 minutes. Turn the heat down a bit more, add butter and simmer for another 5 minutes.

Serves 4

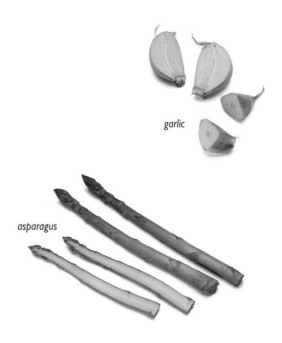

garlic

asparagus

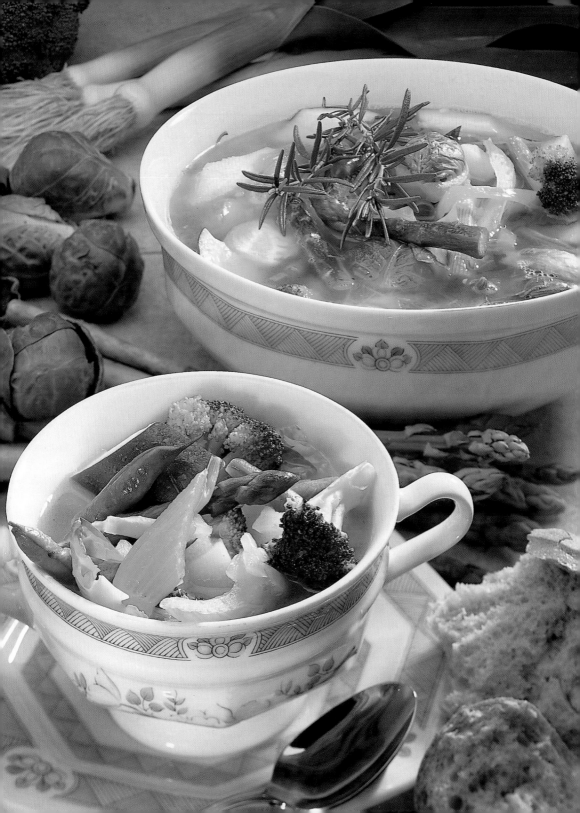

Mushroom Soup with Bread Dumplings

This Bavarian-style soup would have pleased Father Kneipp. Its simplicity is contrasted by its multitude of health benefits. The mushrooms alone, offer a long list of healing properties. And the taste is both unique and worldly.

I lb (450 g) **Portobello mushrooms, in ¼" (5 mm) slices**

1/2 lb (225 g) **white mushrooms, cut in ¼" (5 mm) slices**

2 tbsp **extra-virgin olive oil**

I cup (240 g) **white onion, diced**

3 cloves **garlic, minced**

¼ cup (120 g) **celery root (or celery), diced**

½ qt (½ l) **vegetable stock or water**

Pinch cayenne pepper

½ tsp **ground nutmeg**

3 tbsp **kefir**

Sea salt and freshly ground pepper to taste

I tbsp **organic butter**

2 tsp **fresh thyme leaves**

Bread Dumplings:

4 cups (450 g) **whole wheat bread, cut in I" (2.5 cm) cubes**

½ cup (125 ml) **warm milk or water**

I **free-range egg**

2 tbsp **green onion, chopped**

Dumplings: Heat milk, pour over the bread and mix thoroughly. Let the bread absorb all the milk. Add the egg and onion and mix again. Let it set for 10 minutes. Portion into 1"-diameter balls and place in a 1 quart (1 liter) of salted boiling water. You'll know the dumplings are cooked, when they float up to the top (about 7 to 10 minutes). Turn the heat off and let sit in the water until soup is ready.

Soup: Scrape the brown spores from the insides of the Portobello mushrooms. This will prevent the soup from getting too dark. In a large pot, heat the oil over medium and add the onion, garlic and celery and sauté for 5 minutes, or until soft. Add all of the mushrooms and sauté for another 2 minutes. Add vegetable broth, cayenne and nutmeg and season with salt and pepper. Cover and simmer for 8 to 10 minutes.

Place the soup in a blender and blend until smooth. Add kefir and blend again. Return the soup to the pot, add the butter and thyme and let sit for 2 minutes. Serve with the dumplings.

Serves 4

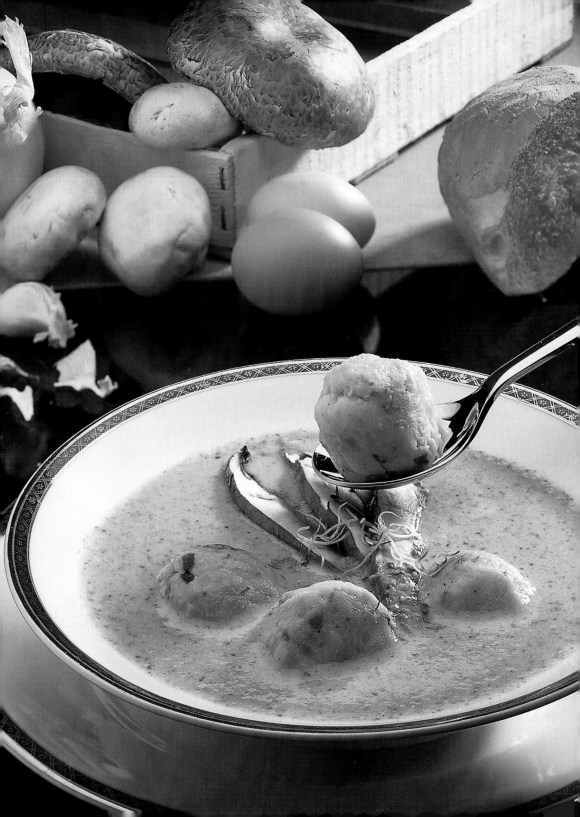

Multigrain Soy Bread

With this hearty recipe, you can enjoy your nutritious grains and protein at the same time. Father Kneipp did not have the luxury of a breadmaker. If you do, simply add the following ingredients as your breadmaker manual suggests and bake on the 3-dough cycle, if you have the option. If you want to make this bread the old-fashioned way, follow the directions below.

1 ¼ cups (310 ml) **warm water**

1 tbsp **honey**

1 tbsp **sunflower or pistachio oil**

1 cup (250 ml) **whole wheat flour**

1 cup (250 ml) **bread flour**

⅓ cup (80 ml) **soy flour**

1 tbsp **nutritional yeast**

¾ cup (185 ml) **multigrain cereal**

2 tbsp **gluten flour**

2 tsp **sea salt**

2 tsp **active dry yeast**

Dissolve yeast (both types) and honey in ¼ cup warm water until yeast foams. Sift all the flours and mix with the salt. Add the remaining water (1 cup), and the yeast mixture, to the flour. Add all remaining ingredients and work the dough with your hands until all ingredients are well combined and dough is smooth with an elastic consistency. Put dough in a bowl, cover with a kitchen towel and set aside for at least 30 minutes at room temperature, or until dough doubles in size.

Grease a bread pan with butter and dust with either flour or cornmeal. Place the dough in the bread pan and bake in preheated oven at 380°F (190°C) for 35 to 40 minutes, or until golden brown. Bake the bread on the top oven rack. Bread is baked when a wooden skewer poked in the middle of it comes out dry.

Makes a 1 ½-pound loaf

Put a bowl of water in the oven with the bread. This will keep the bread moist and will also help to circulate an even temperature in the oven. If you want an extra crispy crust, sprinkle cold water on the top of the loaf, half way through the baking time.

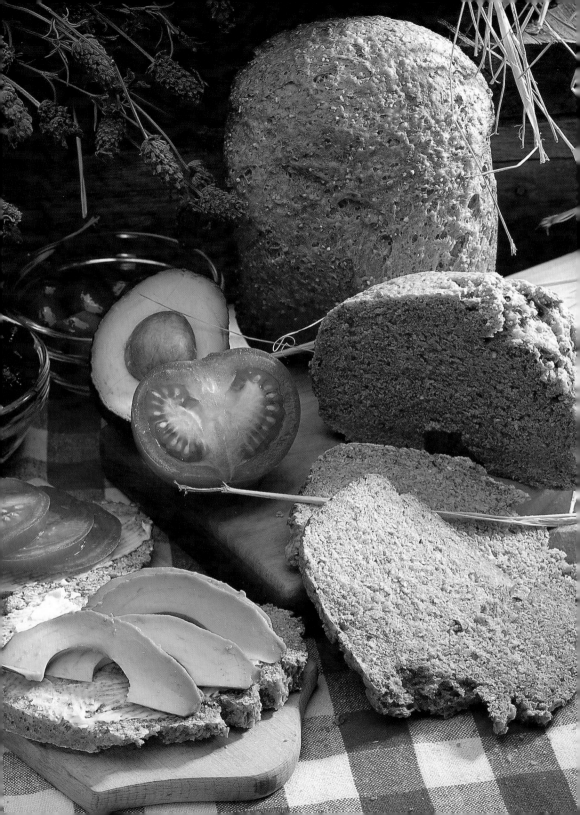

Grilled Vegetables with Quinoa

1 cup (450 g) **quinoa grains**
(or Kamut)

2 tbsp **organic butter**

¼ cup (60 g) **onion, diced**

2 **cloves, minced**

1 tbsp **fresh rosemary,
chopped**

1 tsp **fennel seed**

**Sea salt and freshly
ground pepper to taste**

½ lb (225 g) **baby carrots,
peeled**

3 tbsp **extra-virgin
olive oil**

1 **zucchini, cut in** ½"
(1 cm) **slices**

1 **eggplant, cut in** ½"
(1 cm) **slices**

1 **red bell pepper,
cut in half**

1 **yellow bell pepper,
cut in half**

5 **cloves garlic, whole**

**Sprig of fresh rosemary
for garnish**

2 tbsp **green onion,
chopped for garnish**

Soak the quinoa in water overnight, at room temperature. Rinse the quinoa in a strainer. In a medium pot, place the quinoa and 2 cups (480 ml) with water. Cook, uncovered, on medium heat for 20 minutes or until tender and all the water is evaporated. In a frying pan heat 1 tablespoon of the butter on low heat and sauté onion and minced garlic until soft. Add the quinoa, rosemary and fennel seed, season with salt and pepper and remaining butter.

Brush the garlic and all the vegetables (except for the carrots) with oil, season with salt and pepper and place on a cookie sheet. Roast in oven at 380°F (200°C), turning once until both sides are golden brown (approx 10 minutes). In the meantime, in a large pot, blanch carrots in ½ quart (½ liter) of boiling, salted water for 4 minutes.

To serve, place a pile of quinoa in the center of each plate and arrange the vegetables around it.

Serves 2

garlic

Suggestion:
If you'd like a dressing or sauce for your vegetables, mix the following and drizzle on top once served.
1 tbsp balsamic vinegar
1 tbsp freshly squeezed lemon juice
3 tbsp cold-pressed flax seed oil

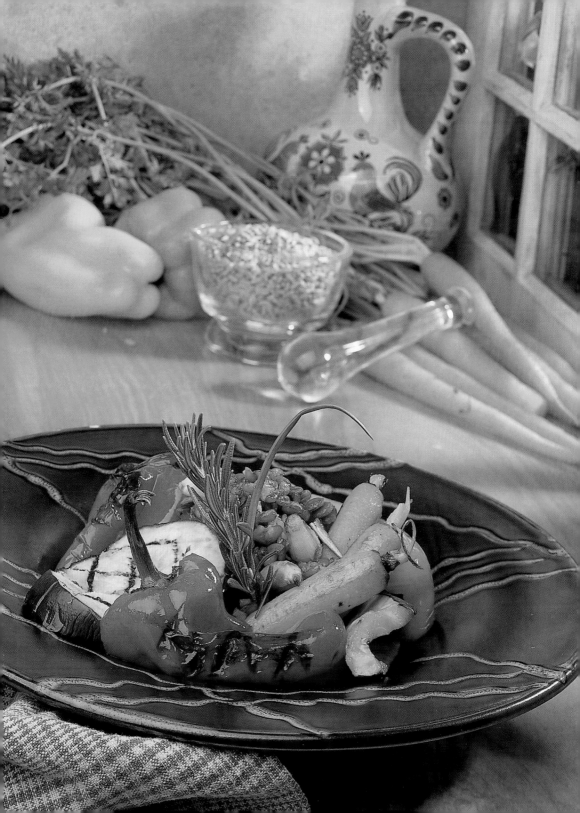

Angelé, Karl-Heinz. Your Daily Health Care with Kneipp. Translated by Judith M. Mariafai and Jane A. Storck. Bad Wörishofen, Kneipp Verlag, 1980.

Bachmann, Robert and German Schleimkofer. Die Kneipp Wassertherapie-Praktische Anleitungen. [Direction for Practical Water Therapy]. Mindelheim, SACHON, 1987.

Burghardt, Ludwig. Helfer der Menschheit Sebastian Kneipp. [Friend of Mankind: Sebastian Kneipp]. Bad Wörishofen, Kneipp Verlag, 1988.

Froehlich, Hans Horst. Der Naturgarten des Sebastian Kneipp. [The Nutrient Garden of Sebastian Kneipp]. Würzburg, Sebastian Kneipp Gesundheitsmittel Verlag, 1993.

Gursche, Siegfried. Encylopedia of Natural Healing. Burnaby, BC: alive books, 1997.

Kneipp, Sebastian. Aus meinem Leben Selbstbiographie. [My Life: A Biography]. Augsburg, Druck Presse, 1891; Bad Wörishofen, Stamm Kneipp Verein, 1979.

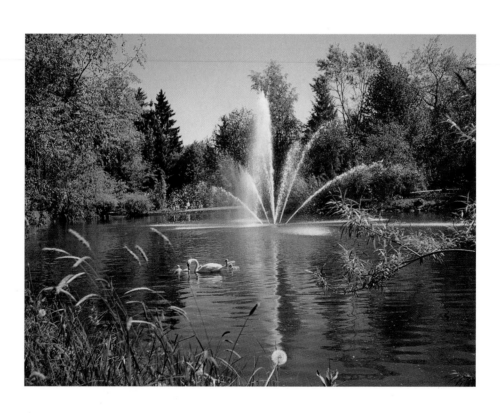

sources

Axel Kraft int.USA Inc.
Fort Lauderdale, Fl.33301 USA
Telephone: 954-942-9038 or 1-800-667-7864

Bad Woerishofer Kraeuterhaus Schweiger
Kneipp wrappers, tubs, socks/all hardware
Suedweg 10, D-86825 Bad Woerishofen Germany
Telephone: 001-49-8247-90180
Fax 001-49-8247-90181
e-mail: info@kraeuterhaus-schweiger.de

"bellmira" products:
Axel Kraft Int. Ltd.,
Aurora, Ontario L4G 3V1 CANADA
Telephone: 905-841-6840
Fax 905-841-6841

Kneipp Corporation of America
105-107 Stonehurst Ct.,
Northvale, NJ 07647 USA
Information Line: 1-800-937-4372
Telephone: (201) 750-0600
Fax: (201) 750-2070

MUNASA INC., Kneipp Distribution Canada
1210 Markham Road, Unit 3
Scarborough, Ontario
M1H 3B3
Telephone: (416) 438-4301
Fax: (416) 438-8658

**Purity Life Health Products Ltd.
(WELEDA Products)**
6 Commerce Crescent,
Acton, Ontario L7J 2X3 CANADA
Telephone: 001-519-853-3511
Fax 001-519-853-4660

WELEDA Inc.
P.O. Box 249,
175 North Route 9W
Congers, NY 10920
Telephone: 914-268-8572
Fax 914-268-8574 or 1-800-241-1030

First published in 2000 by
alive books
7436 Fraser Park Drive
Burnaby BC V5J 5B9
(604) 435–1919
1–800–661–0303

© 2000 by *alive books*

Artwork:
  Liza Novecoski
  Terence Yeung
  Raymond Cheung
Food Styling/Recipe Development:
  Fred Edrissi
Photography:
  Edmond Fong (recipe photos)
  Siegfried Gursche
Photo Editing:
  Sabine Edrissi-Bredenbrock
Editing:
  Sandra Tonn
  Donna Dawson

Canadian Cataloguing in
Publication Data

Roeder, Giselle
  Healing with Water

(alive natural health guides, 11
ISSN 1490-6503)
ISBN 1-55312-011-6

Printed in Canada

Revolutionary Health Books

alive Natural Health Guides

Each 64-page book focuses on a single subject, is written in easy-to-understand language and is lavishly illustrated with full color photographs.

New titles will be published every month in each of the four series.

Self Help Guides

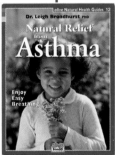

Healthy Recipes

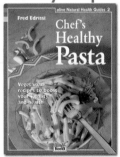

Healing Foods & Herbs

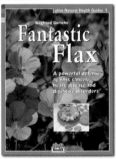

Lifestyle & Alternative Treatments

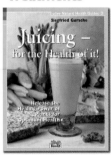

other titles to follow:

- Nature's Own Candida Cure
- Natural Treatment for Chronic Fatigue Syndrome
- Fibromyalgia Be Gone!
- Heart Disease: Save Your Heart Naturally

other titles to follow:

- Baking with the Bread Machine
- Baking Bread: Delicious, Quick and Easy
- Healthy Breakfasts
- Desserts
- Smoothies and Other Healthy Drinks

other titles to follow:

- Calendula: The Healthy Skin Helper
- Ginkgo Biloba: The Good Memory Herb
- Rhubarb and the Heart
- Saw Palmetto: The Key to Prostate Health
- St. John's Wort: Sunshine for Your Soul

other titles to follow:

- Maintain Health with Acupuncture
- The Complete Natural Cosmetics Book
- Breast Health Naturally
- Magnetic Therapy and Natural Healing
- Sauna: Your Way to Better Health

Vancouver
Canada

Great gifts at an amazingly affordable price **$9.95 Cdn / $8.95 US / £8.95 UK**

alive Natural Health Guides are available in health and nutrition centers and in bookstores. For information or to place orders please dial 1-800-663-6513